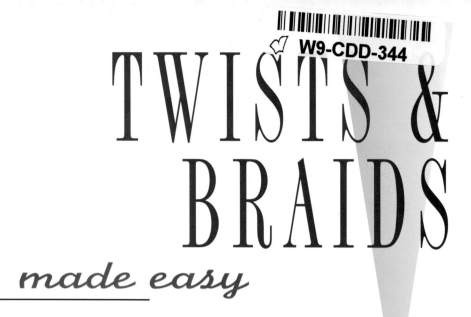

TWISTS & BRAIDS
made easy

Writer, Hair Designer, and Makeup Artist:
Mary Beth Janssen-Fleischman

Publications International, Ltd.

Mary Beth Janssen-Fleischman is a hair and beauty industry professional with film and television credits and extensive experience with consumer and trade magazines. She has contributed to magazines including *Modern Salon, American Salon, Harper's Bazaar,* and *Coiffure de Paris.* She has served as contributing writer and hair designer for numerous hairstyle books including *Beautiful Braids* and *Pony Tails and Other Hair Designs.*

Technical Assistant to Mary Beth Janssen-Fleischman: Barbara Kauth
Photography by David Puffer
Photo Assistant: Ed Ernst
Props: WITH STYLE: Sally Mauer, Hilary Rose
Models: Royal Model Management: Pamela Berk, Karen Lea, Stephanie Loyola, Laura Truxler; The Models Workshop Studio: Rachel Hebert.

Contents

Introduction

Women and girls with long hair—even hair with long layers—are blessed with opportunities to create hair designs that run the gamut from stunning and glamorous to pretty and casual. They can twist it, roll it, braid it, curl it, sweep it back, arrange it to frame the face, accessorize it—so many exciting options exist!

Best of all, the various design techniques are easy to master. It's only a myth that short hair gets you out of the house faster in the morning. Rolling, twisting, braiding, and other techniques on the following pages are all relatively simple and straightforward—and the results can be beautiful.

Once you become comfortable with a particular technique, think about the many possibilities for it and how you might adapt it to different types of hair—perhaps for a family member or a close friend. You've got the best of both worlds when you can combine techniques to create your own designs.

Before getting started on individual styles, review the basic techniques, tools, and accessories that make hair designing a breeze!

Techniques

The Inverted Ponytail

The inversion technique, which basically turns a ponytail upside down and inside out, is accomplished using an easy-to-handle inversion tool. The result is an elegant twisted roll effect on either side of the ponytail.

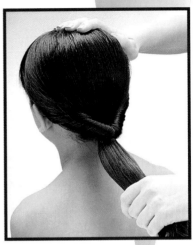

The Inverted Ponytail

The Twist

Individual sections can be twisted independently, or two sections can be twisted together. The resulting pattern resembles a rope. This technique can be performed on the free ends of a ponytail. Use small sections and twist tightly for a defined effect, or use large sections and twist loosely for a softer, more voluminous look.

Twists may be done in partial areas or throughout the head. When a very large section of hair is rolled while twisting along an area of the head, a twisted roll results. When placed vertically at the back of the head, it is called a classic French twist.

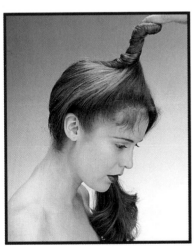

The Twist

The Roll

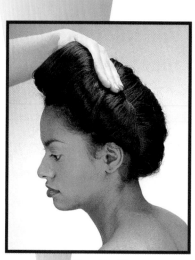

Hair that is rolled, overlapping upon itself, has a beautiful, full shape, without the directional influence a twisted roll has. Use hair fillers (see "Tools and Accessories") to create the desired volume if the hair does not have enough density or is simply too fine.

The Roll

The Braid

The basic braid is either the three-strand overbraid or the three-strand underbraid. In overbraiding, the outside strands are crossed over the center strand. The pattern is reversed in underbraiding: Outside strands are crossed under the center strand. In overbraiding, it appears as if the strands originate from the outside and move into the center. In underbraiding, the strands seem to move from the inside of the braid pattern toward the outside.

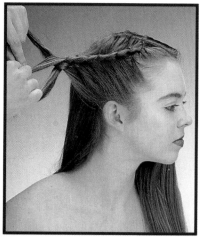

Asymmetrical Braid

An asymmetrical braiding technique involves picking up hair from along the scalp on the hairline side only. This creates a more mobile free braid; whether underbraided or overbraided, it has a unique pattern.

6

Four-strand braiding techniques result in more intricate patterns. The technique is a little more involved, but the results are stunning.

The four-strand round braid creates an elaborate design that is chainlike and round in configuration. The technique is mastered quite easily when you follow the basic steps: The outside strands are brought under the two inside strands and back over one of them.

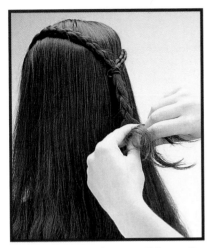

Four-strand round braid

With the chain braid, outside strands weave across the width of the braid, alternating from side to side. This braid is wide and flat, with an interwoven texture.

The designs you can create with these braiding techniques are endless. You can braid all the hair together as one section, or you can braid several smaller sections. If you're braiding several small sections of the hair, try varying

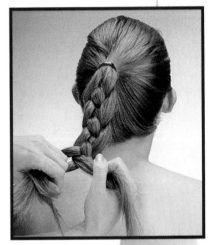

Chain Braid

the braiding technique. Another option is to braid decorative cord or ribbon into the design. The variations are limitless.

7

Tools and Accessories

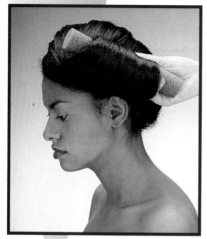
Hair filler

Hairpins and bobby pins come in a variety of lengths and colors. Long, large bobby pins are especially effective when pinning larger shapes or working on thick hair. Hairpins are used where a more delicate part of the design requires pinning for hold and a bobby pin won't fit into the area being worked on.

Coated elastic bands provide one of the easiest and safest ways to fasten hair. Repeated use of uncoated elastic bands may cause hair breakage. Using a coated band to secure ponytails and the ends of a braid or twist design reduces wear and tear on your hair.

Hair fillers help create rolls. Choose the type based on the amount of volume you want. Simply roll the hair around the filler from the ends to the scalp and pin in place to secure.

French twist comb

The French twist comb holds your French twist decoratively, yet firmly in place. After creating your rolled French twist, don't use hairpins—just insert the teeth of the comb into the seam area. The comb should catch the hair between the base and the rolled formation, holding the twist firmly in place.

The crochet technique pulls hair up and away from the face. A crochet hook is used to loop and pull decorative cording through the hair design in a woven pattern.

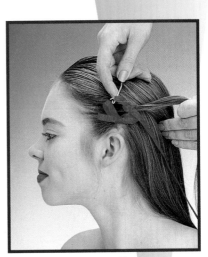
Crochet technique

Hints and Tips

Damp or dry? You must decide whether to perform the technique on damp or dry hair. Damp hair sometimes gives you control in managing stray ends or layers of hair. Adding a light spray gel to the dampened hair provides added control. Working with dry hair, you achieve effects that are soft and have greater volume. If you choose to work on dry hair, a light misting of water as you work helps control flyaways.

Gels control hair lengths, too. You can apply gel to all of the hair before you braid, or, when you want a clean, off-the-face effect, you can apply it just to the hairline where lengths tend to be shorter.

Besides using **hair spray** to hold the finished design in place, try using it in spot areas as you work. Also, if you want to create a soft finish but need to control the hair, spray lightly into the palm of your hand and then smooth over the surface of the hair to control flyaway strands before, during, and after designing.

9

TOUCH OF CLASS
Classic French twist

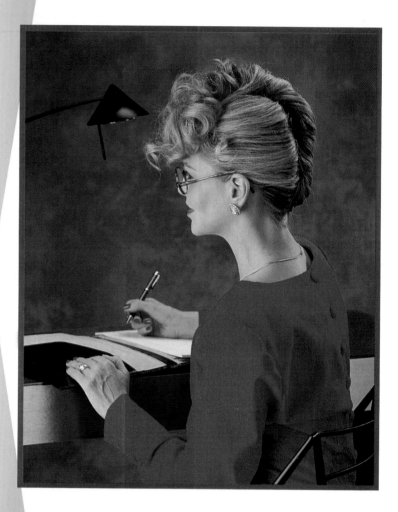

In this classic interpretation of the French twist, the method
used is excellent for shorter as well as longer lengths of hair. It
also lets you make the French twist larger if greater volume is
desired.

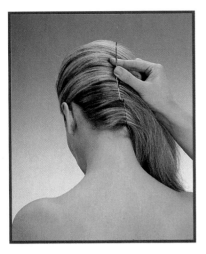

1. Direct hair to the center back from the left side of the head. Brush or comb smoothly, and lightly mist with hair spray as needed. Pin with long hairpins vertically through the back. (Note how the pins are slightly to the right.)

2. Brush the right side toward the center back and begin to turn the hair, starting from the nape upward. The hair is wrapped within itself in a cylindrical twist.

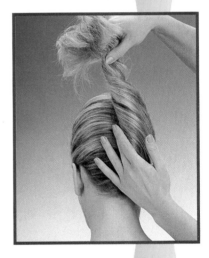

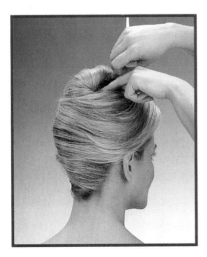

3. Continue twisting the hair upward toward the top of the head. Use a tail comb to tuck any stray ends into the seam of the twist. Tuck the ends into the top of the twist and pin them.

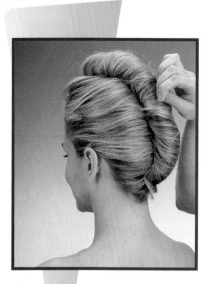

4. Use hairpins to secure along the seam of the twist, inserting them so that one side of the hairpin catches the twist, while the other side catches the scalp hair. (Insert the hairpin upward, then turn it downward to give extra hold.)

5. If the hair is long enough, the French twist can extend further into the top area of the head. Otherwise, the bangs or fringe hair may be curled or arranged and pinned in place.

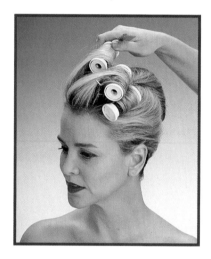

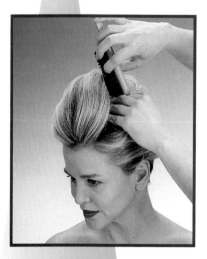

6. If this top hair is long enough and a sleeker look is desired, you may brush the hair back and blend it with the top of the French twist.

TOUCH OF CLASS
Variation

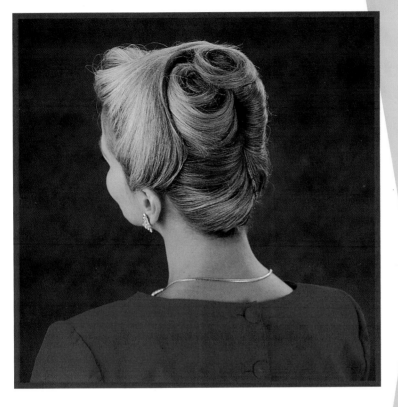

1. Part the hair down the center back. Then divide each part again. This will create two back sections and two side sections.

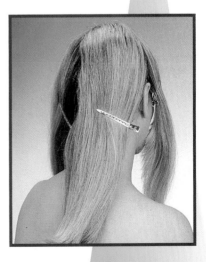

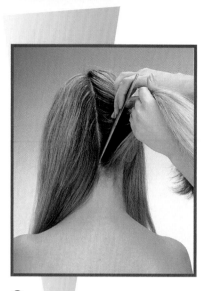

2. Direct one of the back sections up and away from the center and toward one side of the head. Lay the end of a tail comb down the center back. The comb should be angled away from the head.

3. Wrap the free lengths of the back section around the tail of the comb. If lengths are too short, roll the twist from the bottom to the top as outlined in the first design.

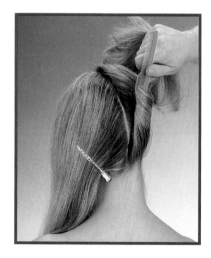

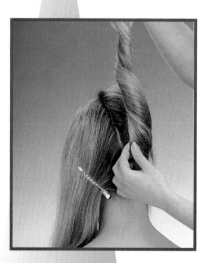

4. Remove the comb and twist the remaining ends in the same direction. Pull the twist upward and fan the twist to balance the vertical roll.

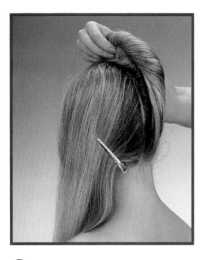

5. Curve the free ends down in a circular formation at the crown and pin to secure.

6. Repeat this technique for the opposite side of the back, this time angling the hair up and sideways in the opposite direction.

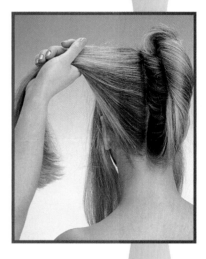

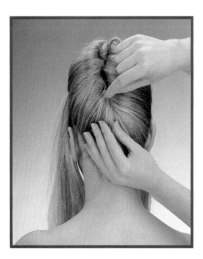

7. Position the tail comb and wrap the ends around it in an upward direction. Remove the comb and twist the remaining ends. Secure the free ends. Pin through the center back, joining the two rolls together at the seam.

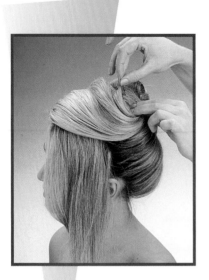

8. Each side section will be crossed over toward its opposite side. Take the right section, brush it back and form a decorative loop with the ends to surround the top left ends of the roll in back.

9. Repeat for the opposite side section. Brush the left side back and across the head toward the top right-side roll. Loop the ends around the top of the back roll and pin in place.

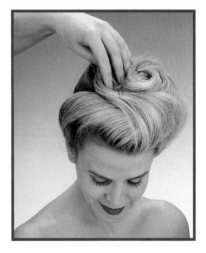

16

QUICK TWIST
Partial French twist

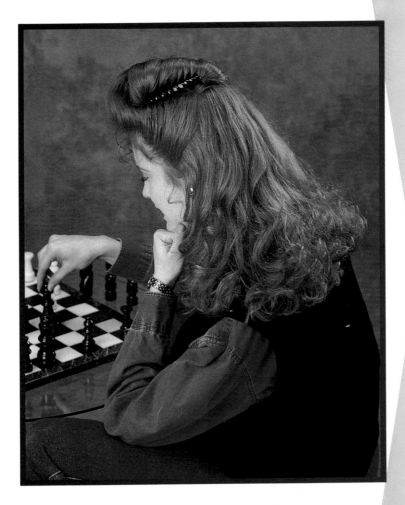

This is the simplest technique for creating a partial French twist

at the crown that contrasts with full, flowing lengths of hair.

This design can be dressy or very casual to fit your different

moods.

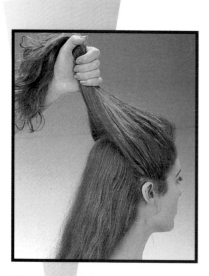

1. Gather the sides together with the crown hair. Direct these lengths up and out from the crown. (If the top front hair is not long enough to twist, you can style it as desired.)

2. Position your hand beneath the gathered hair at the lower crown. Turn the hair over the hand to begin the French twist.

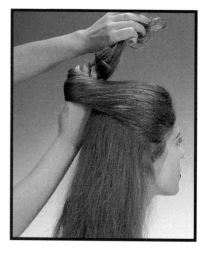

3. Twist the hair up to the ends. Then turn the hair around and under the twist.

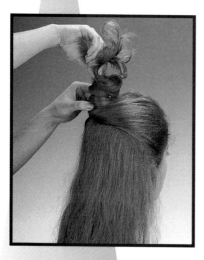

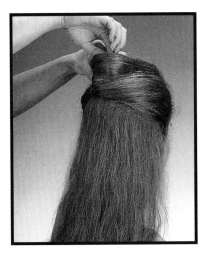

4. Depending on the length of the twisted ends, you may need to make more than one turn under the twist. Tuck the ends in to prepare for securing.

5. The twist is secured with a decorative French twist comb specially designed with large, wide-spaced teeth for a firm lock. Make sure that the comb is inserted into both the twist and the smooth hair at the scalp.

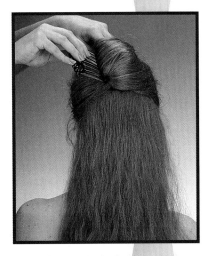

DANGEROUS CURVES
Figure-eight nape chignon

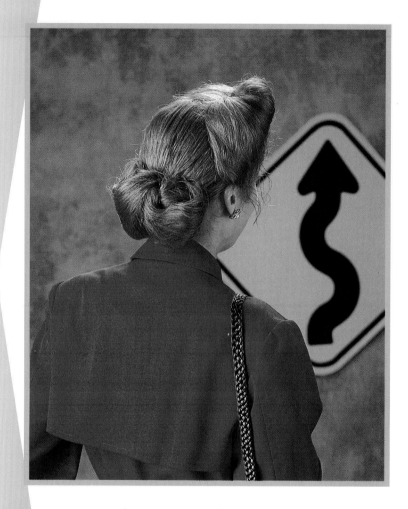

This imaginative, unique design combines a delicate, curved roll in the front area with a looped, or figure-eight, chignon at the nape. The effect is absolutely smashing!

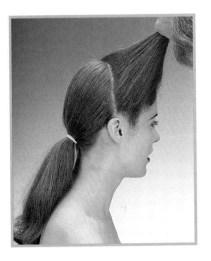

1. Divide the front hair from the back, sectioning from the top of one ear over the head to the top of the other ear. Secure a ponytail at the nape. Bring all hair in the front area up and over toward the top side. Brush hair smooth.

2. The direction that you hold the hair is important in positioning the roll properly. Here, the ends are directed up and out from the top side area. Roll the ends around themselves to begin the roll procedure.

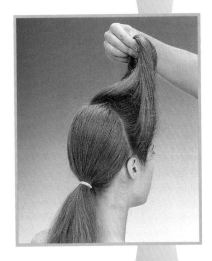

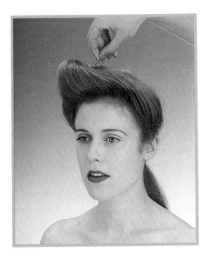

3. Continue to roll the hair around itself toward the scalp. When the hair has been fully rolled, hold the roll in place while you secure it as needed with bobby pins or hairpins. Mist with hair spray for added hold.

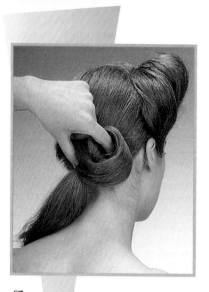

4. Divide the ponytail in half leaving the fastener in place. Back-comb the sections slightly for control in positioning the loops. Form a loop with one section by turning the ends toward the center area of the ponytail.

5. Turn and tuck the ends around the base of the ponytail. Secure these ends through the fastened area of the ponytail with hairpins.

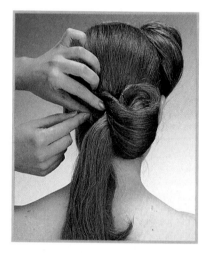

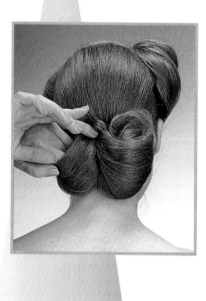

6. Form the opposite section into a loop for the other side of the figure eight. Bring the ends up and around the fastened ponytail and secure with hairpins. Mist with hair spray.

A LA FRANÇAISE
Three twists

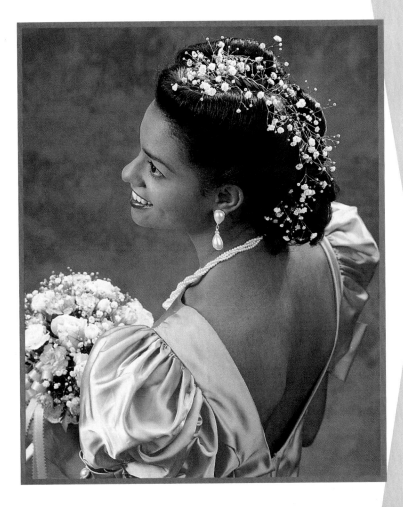

The simple beauty of this design owes as much to its unity of style as to the ease with which it is created. Triple twists create a balance that is stunning, and you can alter the mood with the hair ornaments you choose.

23

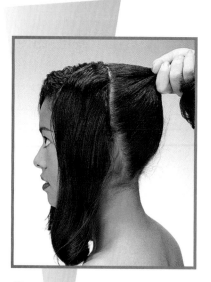

1. Divide the front hair from the back, sectioning from the top of one ear over the head to the top of the other ear. Beginning in the back area, gather the hair up toward the lower crown and hold it in a ponytail.

2. Twist the ponytail down toward the nape into a cylindrical twist. The ends can hang down naturally for a casual look, or they may be tucked in.

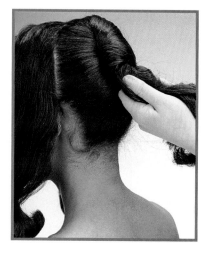

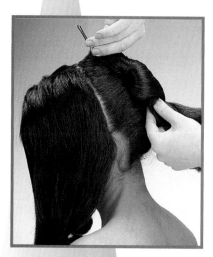

3. Pin along the seam area and into the ends of the twist to secure it.

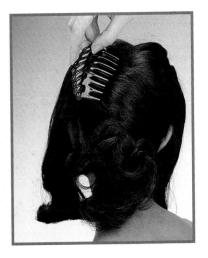

4. You may also use a French twist comb, specially made to hold the thicker elongated twist shape. Insert along the seam area of the twist, securing the twist and the scalp hair together.

5. The same technique is used on both sides for the remaining hair. Divide this hair in half (right and left), and on the right side direct the hair up and out from the top side area.

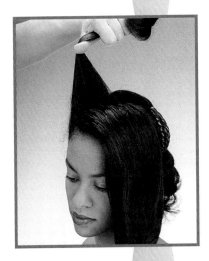

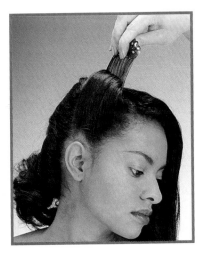

6. With the thumb and index finger, turn the hair ends down toward the scalp. Use bobby pins as necessary. Secure with a decorative hair comb. Repeat on the opposite side, securing the twist with a comb.

A LA FRANÇAISE
Variation

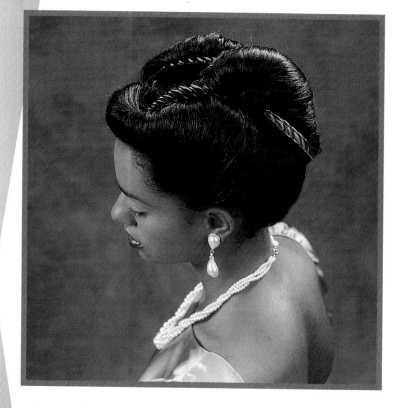

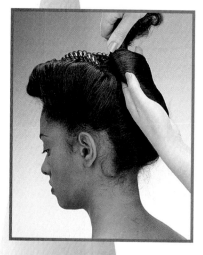

1. Divide the hair into two sections and repeat steps 5 and 6 from the first design. Grasp a ponytail at the back area and twist upward. Place your hand underneath the twisted ponytail. Then fold the twist over and under your hand.

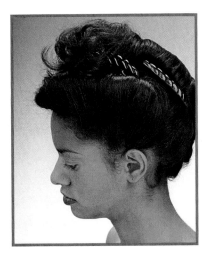

2. Keep tension on the ponytail by twisting close to the head. The ends may be left loose and full after you've pinned along the top area to secure the twist.

3. To create a more structured style, you can tuck the ends under the twist at the crown and pin in place.

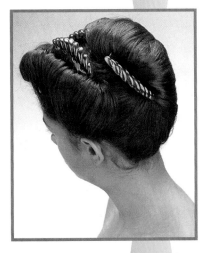

BERIBBONED BEAUTY
The ribbon weave

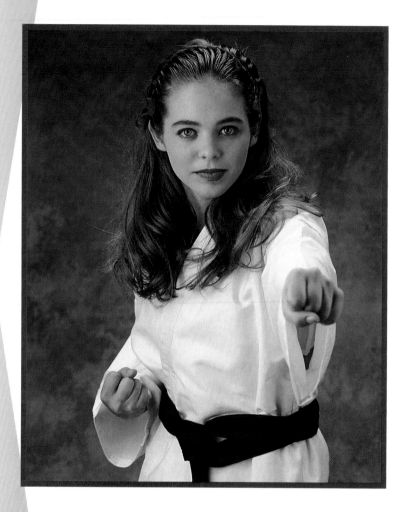

This design is simple and fun to make. Whether the look is sporty or romantic, the results are exquisitely flattering. A much better way to bring hair away from the face than using barrettes, hairpins, or combs!

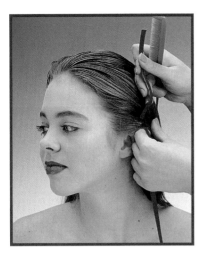

1. Direct all hair off the face. (Misting with water helps control strands as you work.) Beginning above the ear on one side of the head, scale out a half-inch of hair and insert one end of a yard of ribbon behind the strand of hair.

2. Tie a bow with the short end and long end of the ribbon. Remember to work closely to the scalp to avoid lifting the hair up and away.

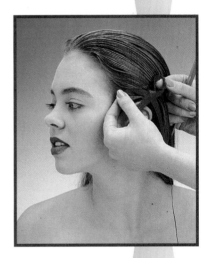

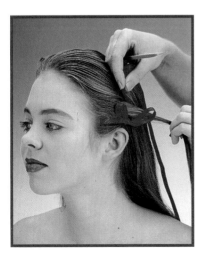

3. Scale out another small section of hair, directly above the previous section, and pull the ribbon underneath it.

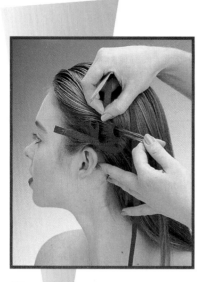

4. Next, direct the ribbon around the same strand, looping the ribbon. Pull to maintain control and smoothness. This will be the procedure used throughout.

5. Continue up and over the head, aiming for the top of the ear on the other side. Try to work with strands of equal size, and maintain consistency in loops and tension for best results.

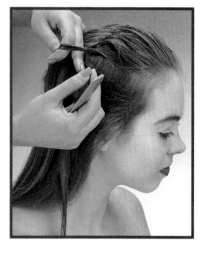

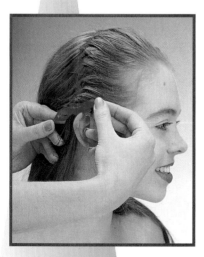

6. When you reach the final section, make another bow and cut off the excess ribbon. Soft tendrils of hair may be left free around the forehead; back lengths may be curled or left straight.

BERIBBONED BEAUTY
Variation

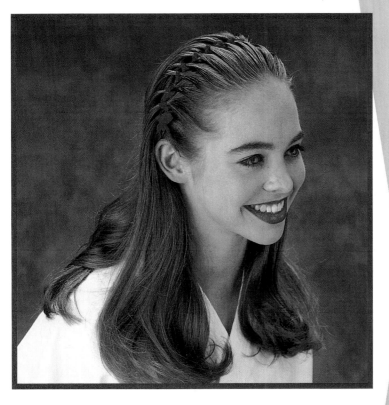

1. Begin the technique in the first design, but instead of picking up sections and directing the ribbon underneath, direct the end of a crochet hook downward behind the sections of hair. Place the ribbon in the hook.

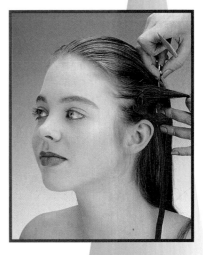

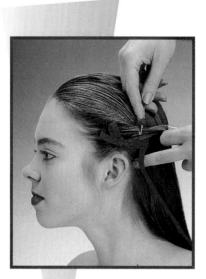

2. Pull the crochet hook up from behind the section of hair to form a loop—but don't pull the long end of the ribbon all the way through. You've now made a small loop; release the ribbon.

3. Extend the hook through the loop and downward to grasp the long end of the ribbon. Secure it in the hook.

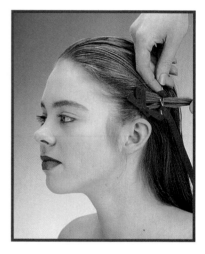

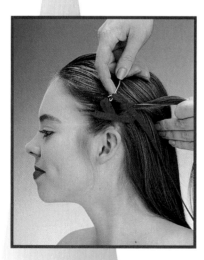

4. Pull this loose end all the way through the loop to form the first crochet loop.

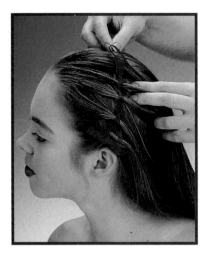

5. Continue sectioning hair to the other side of the head above the ear, performing the crochet technique as you go. Finish off as in the first design.

R emember...
Lightly misting the hair with water helps control the strands as you work.

SMART 'N' SASSY
Asymmetrical rolls

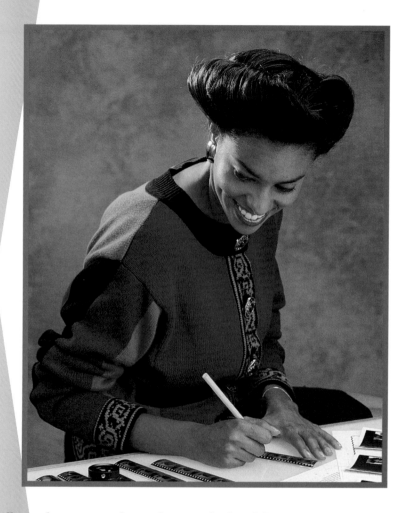

Twisted rolls can be positioned anywhere on the head for
different volume and design emphasis. There are several
variations of the twisted roll—this particular design features an
asymmetrical positioning of rolls.

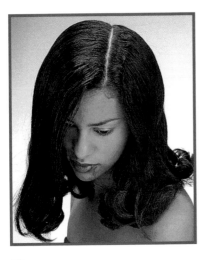

1. Part the hair from front to back, along the side area, curving back to the crown. Begin on the heavier side of the part.

2. Grasp a section of hair and brush it up and out from the top. Place your hand underneath the section of hair, resting the hand against the scalp. Roll the hair around the hand. Pin from behind.

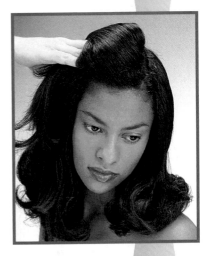

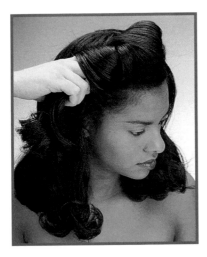

3. Part the next section along the hairline with your fingers. Bring the section upward and roll it over your hand. Comb your fingers through the hair to smooth it. This section of hair will cover the ends from the first section. Pin to secure.

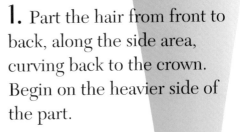

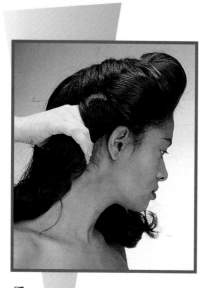

4. Continue to pick up sections as you curve the roll formation downward toward the nape.

5. When you've reached the center back area, pin the hair ends temporarily.

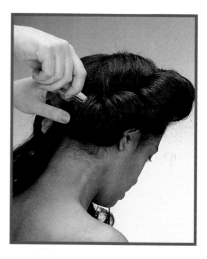

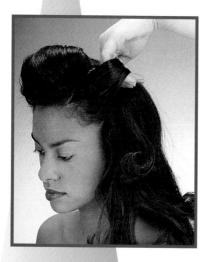

6. Begin the procedure on the opposite side. Comb the hair out on an angle and over your other hand. Roll the section over your hand and pin at the back area to secure.

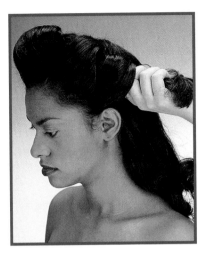

7. Continue the technique of picking up hair from the hairline area, then bringing the lengths up and around the hand. Put a slight backward twist on the hair as you work. Pin as needed to secure.

8. When you reach the back area, pin the ends. If the hair is long enough, form several decorative loops with the ends of the hair, pinning each loop with a hairpin to secure.

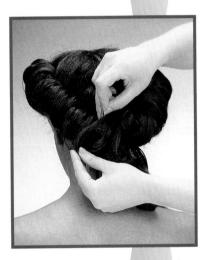

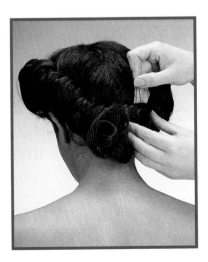

9. Form decorative loops with the ends from the other side to balance and complete the design.

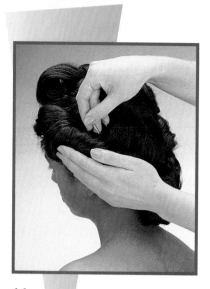

10. If the twisted rolls are heavy, secure them to the scalp hair along the edges.

11. If the hair ends are too short, or if you wish simply to create a sleeker result, finish off the ends of the twisted rolls by turning them back and into the hair design.

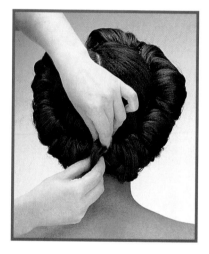

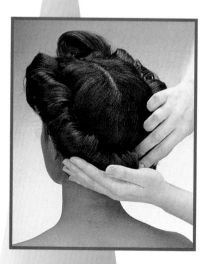

12. Fan out the edges of the roll and secure with pins as needed. Mist with hair spray.

SMART 'N' SASSY
First Variation (with braided hair piece)

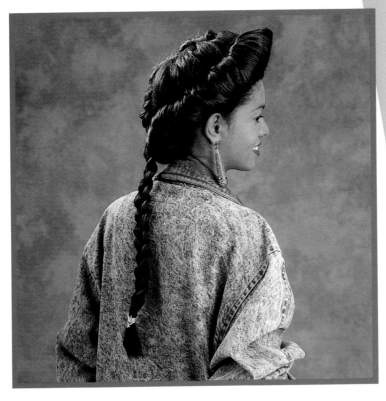

1. Complete the asymmetrical rolls from the first design. Before finishing off the ends of the rolls from both sides, attach a swatch of hair securely at the nape and pin as needed.

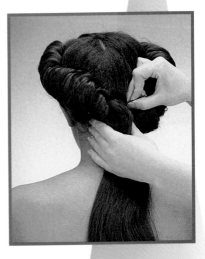

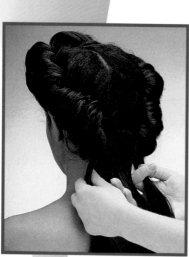

2. To begin the three-strand overbraiding technique, divide the swatch of hair into three equal sections. Hold the left strand with your left hand; hold the other two strands in your right hand—both palms facing upward.

3. Turn your right hand palm down. This will make the right strand automatically switch positions with the center strand. Now, hold two strands in your left hand and one strand in your right, palms facing upward.

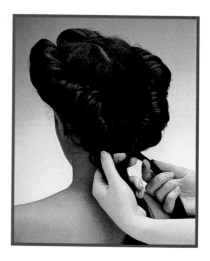

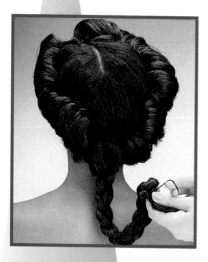

4. Turn your left hand over so the palm faces down. This will make the left strand switch positions with the center strand. Continue overbraiding to the ends and fasten with a **coated** elastic band.

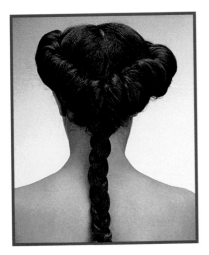

5. Roll the ends of the hair that were pinned out of the way in steps 5 and 8 from the first design. Fan the ends in a rolled formation over the base of the braid attachment and pin to secure.

Remember...
If you're having trouble rolling sections of the hair, back-comb the hair and use hair spray as needed.

SMART 'N' SASSY
Second Variation

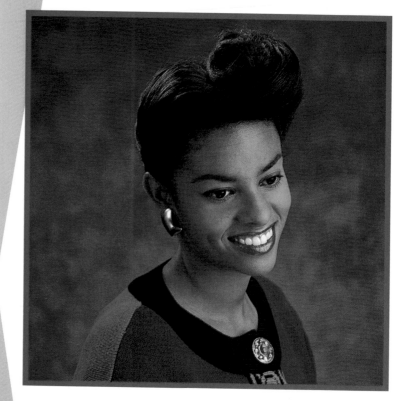

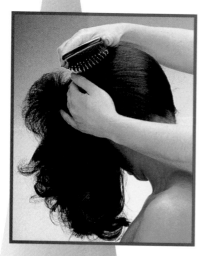

1. Brush all of the hair smoothly to one side of the head. (The hair should be dry for best results.)

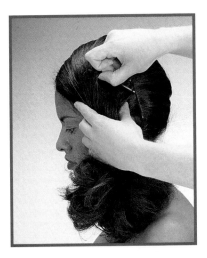

2. When you've determined the position of the roll, place long hairpins vertically along the hair where the roll will be placed.

3. Beginning at the back nape, twist and roll a section of the hair upward. Continue to grasp sections and roll up toward the front of the head. Pin as you work.

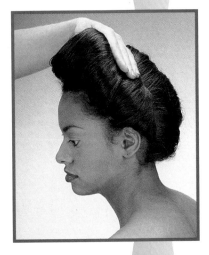

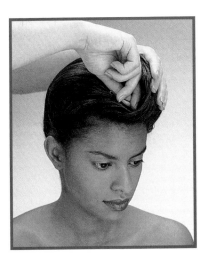

4. When you reach the top front, complete the twisted rolling procedure. Secure the ends in a smooth fashion if a sleeker look is desired or leave them free for a looser texture.

SIMPLY LOVELY
Inverted ponytail

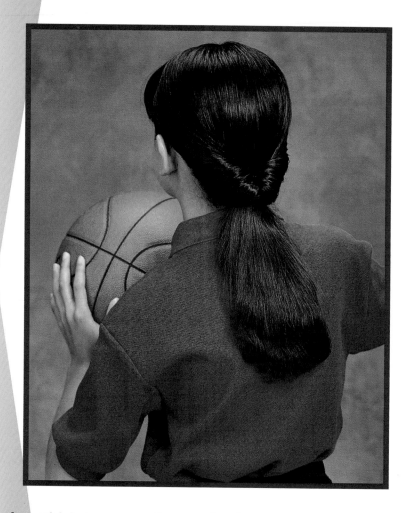

Simple yet beautiful designs are easily created with an inversion technique that turns a basic ponytail upside down and inside out. The inverted ponytail may be positioned with the ends left loose and flowing or curled, braided, or twisted.

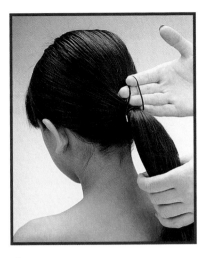

1. Position a ponytail at the back of the head. Fasten it with a **coated** elastic band. (**Caution:** Don't fasten the band too tightly, as the hair needs to be able to move.)

2. Place an inversion tool behind the elastic band of the ponytail. There are many ways to place the tool, each with its own unique result. In this design, we're placing the tool straight up and down for a symmetrical effect.

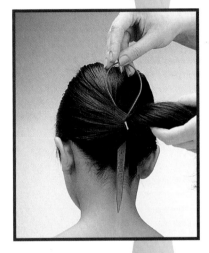

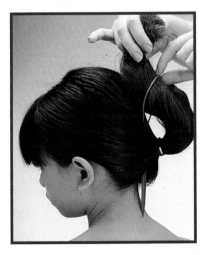

3. Bring the ends of the ponytail up through the loop of the tool. Pull the ponytail through the loop, leaving a little slack to allow the hair to turn more easily.

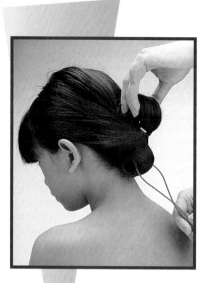

4. Pull the tool down through the hair behind the elastic band. If the tool does not pull through easily, release some tension on the elastic band. As you pull the tool through, the ponytail will follow.

5. Continue to pull the tool down until it and the hair come out below the band. The inversion tool will pull free from the ponytail.

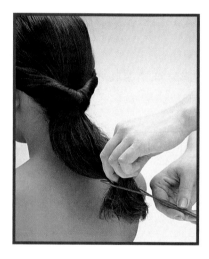

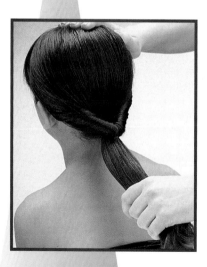

6. Secure the hair design by pulling down on the ends. (If the inverted ponytail feels too loose, separate the ends into two strands and pull into opposite directions.)

SIMPLY LOVELY
Variation

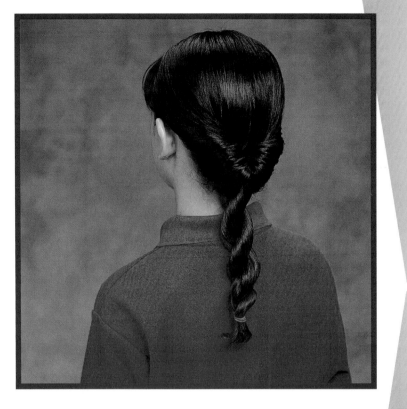

1. Create the basic inverted ponytail from the first design. Separate the hair into two strands. Cross the right strand over the left.

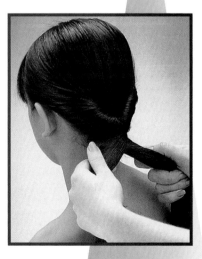

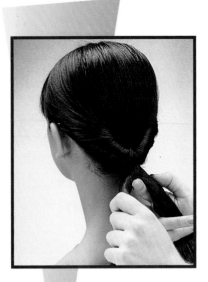

2. Twist the strand that is now on the left clockwise. Put the index finger of the right hand, palm up, into the crossover area of the two strands, meanwhile maintaining tension on the twisted strand.

3. The right hand will turn the two strands over each other in a clockwise direction. Note how turning the hand from a palm-up to a palm-down position makes a two-strand twist.

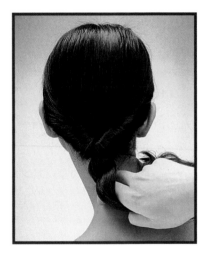

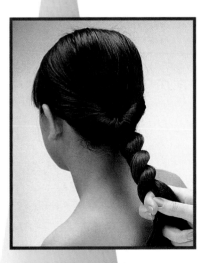

4. Continue twisting the left strand clockwise, then placing the right index finger with palm up, followed by turning the hand clockwise to a palm-down position. Fasten the ends together with a **coated** elastic band.

SMOOTH CONTROL
Partial inversion

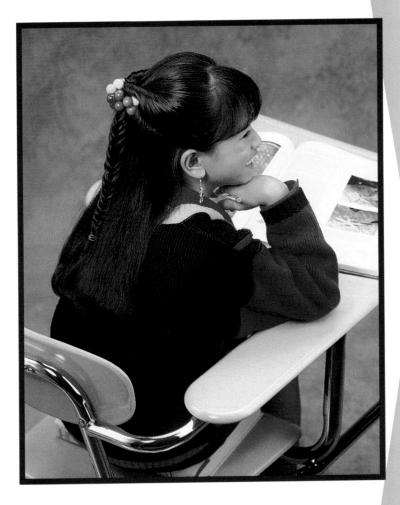

The partial inversion design, combining smoothly controlled hair with a very pretty look, works well for those who want long, flowing hair coupled with control over varying interior lengths.

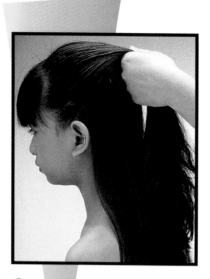

1. Gather hair from the sides and the crown. Direct all lengths to the crown of the head and fasten with a **coated** elastic band to create a ponytail.

2. Use the basic inversion technique for the ponytail. Place the inversion tool behind the elastic band in a vertical position. Insert the ends of the ponytail up and through the loop of the tool.

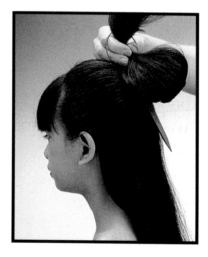

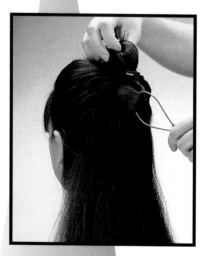

3. Pull on the tool to direct the ponytail behind and through the area beneath the elastic band. The tool will pull the ponytail through and release it to create an inverted ponytail above loose, flowing nape hair.

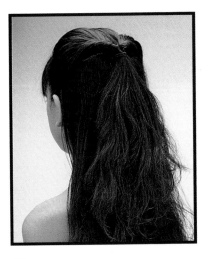

4. The ends may remain loose for a soft, flowing look. You can also create a twisted or braided variation on the ponytail for a more styled design.

5. Here, we're performing the two-strand overlap technique. Divide the ponytail in half and hold the two strands in the left hand. Using your right hand, separate a small section of hair from the right strand.

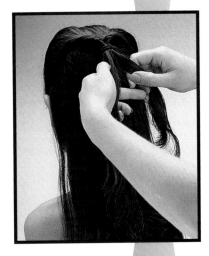

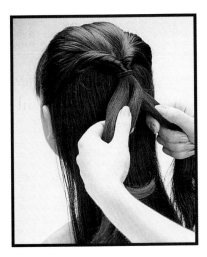

6. Cross this section over to the left strand so that it becomes a part of the left strand. Run your right hand down the length of hair to smooth the strands together.

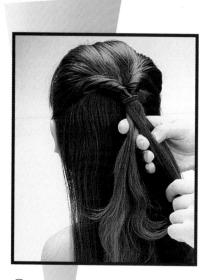

7. Move the two strands to your right hand and hold them. Using your left hand, separate a small section of hair from the left strand and cross it over to the right strand so that it becomes a part of the right strand.

8. Alternating from the right strand to the left strand, continue separating small sections from each strand and crossing them over to the other strand until you reach the end of the ponytail.

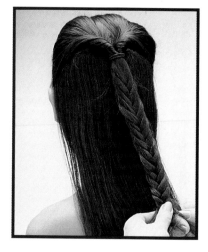

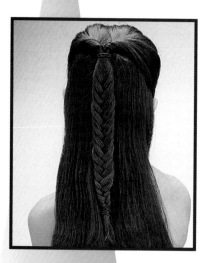

9. Secure the end with a **coated** elastic band. Add ornamentation as desired. The free ends of the loose, flowing hair may be left to fall straight, or they may be curled.

CLASSIC BEAUTY
Inverted ponytail with classic chignon

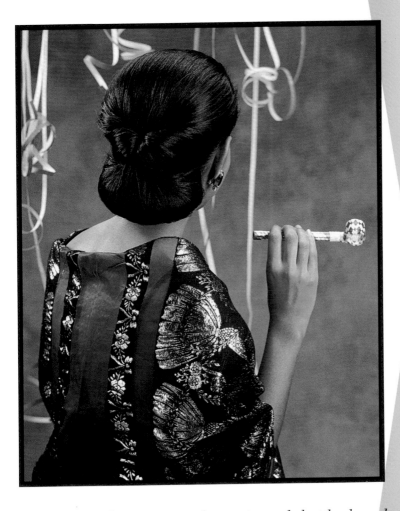

In this design, the inversion technique is coupled with a looped

chignon at the nape, creating a twisted roll effect above a

polished-shell pattern. It's perfect for either long or mid-length

hair and does double-duty as a daytime or evening style.

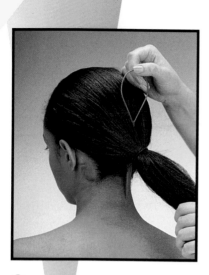

1. Gather the hair at the back of the head and fasten with a **coated** elastic band. Use an inversion tool to create an inverted ponytail: Insert the inversion tool behind the elastic band of the ponytail in a straight vertical position.

2. Bring the ends of the ponytail up through the loop of the tool. Pull the ponytail through the loop, leaving a little slack.

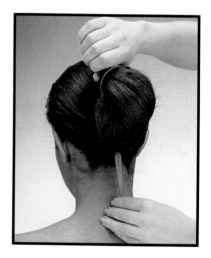

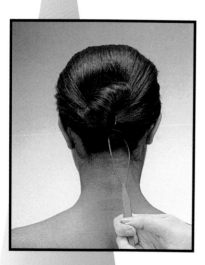

3. Pull the tool down through the hair behind the elastic band. (If the tool does not pull through easily, loosen the tension on the elastic band.)

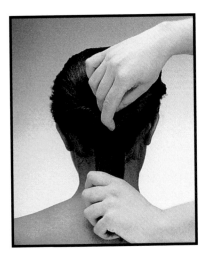

4. Continue to pull the tool down until it and the hair come out below the band. The inversion tool will pull free from the ponytail. Secure the design by pulling down on the ends of the ponytail.

5. Now, divide the ponytail into two strands and pull outward in opposite directions to tighten the rolls created by the inversion technique.

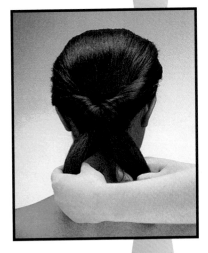

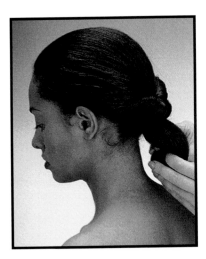

6. Comb the ends of the ponytail back together, then turn the ends under to begin rolling the ponytail toward the scalp.

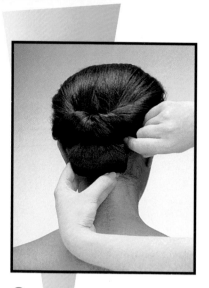

7. Continue to roll the hair toward the scalp. Fasten the rolled hair with bobby pins to secure it.

8. Fan the outside edges of the fastened roll.

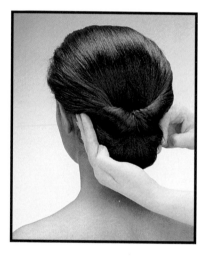

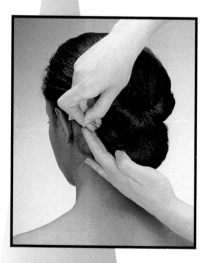

9. Secure these edges with hairpins on either side to hold the fan shape in position. A light misting of hair spray ensures extra hold.

TEXTURAL INTEREST
Double inversion

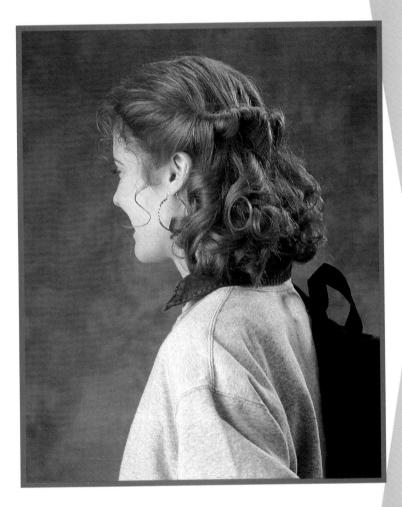

This versatile and attractive design, perfect for any occasion, is
a delightful mix of textures. The sleek top and sides contrast
with the curled ends of two ponytails inverted at the back of the
head.

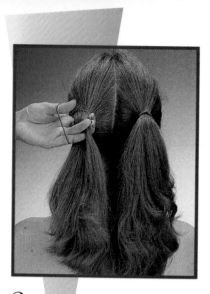

1. Position two ponytails side by side at the back of the head. Fasten them loosely, placing the **coated** elastic bands about two inches from the scalp. This will allow for the double inversion.

2. Use the basic inversion technique on one of the ponytails: Insert the inversion tool behind the ponytail and direct the ends of the ponytail up and through the loop of the tool.

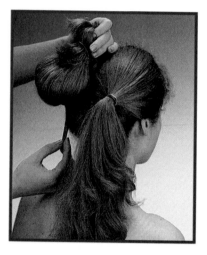

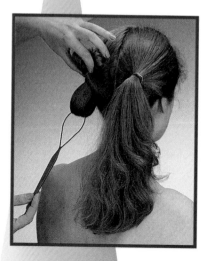

3. Pull the tool through the area behind the elastic band. The tool and ponytail will emerge from underneath the fastened area. Repeat the inversion procedure on the second ponytail.

58

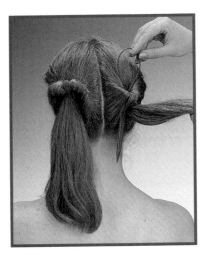

4. Perform the inversion technique a second time on both ponytails, making sure that the tool follows the same path. This double turnaround winds the hair tighter and higher, creating a twisted roll effect.

5. The ends of the hair can be treated in a variety of ways. Here, we're curling the ends, creating a very feminine flounce.

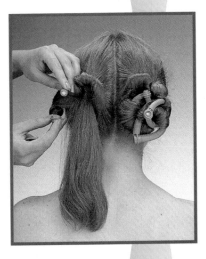

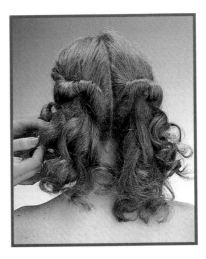

6. Finger-comb the curled ends for a more defined texture, or brush through the hair to create a softer, more diffused look. Mist with hair spray as a finishing touch.

POLISHED SOPHISTICATION
Inverted ponytail with crown chignon

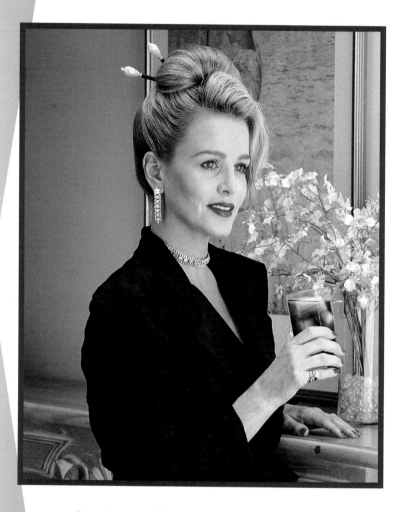

The look is upswept and sophisticated! Here, the inversion
technique is reversed—the ponytail is pulled toward the top of
the head, then shaped into a chignon at the crown for fullness.

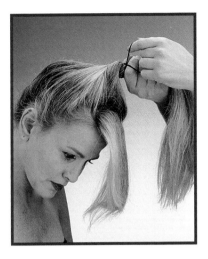

1. Direct all the lengths up to the crown. Bangs or fringe hair may remain loose and flowing. Twist the ponytail before fastening it with a **coated** elastic band.

2. Insert the inversion tool through the area behind the elastic band, going from the back of the head toward the front. The loop will be positioned behind the ponytail.

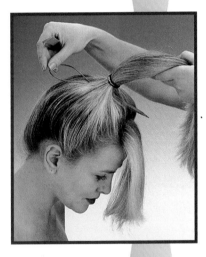

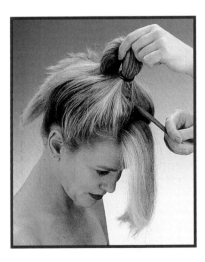

3. Direct the ends of the ponytail through the loop of the tool. Begin pulling the inversion tool, with the ponytail caught inside it, through the area behind the elastic band. Loosen the elastic band, if necessary.

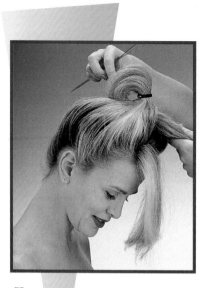

4. The tool and hair will emerge at the top front area of the head. The ends will be used to create the chignon effect.

5. Begin rolling the ends of the hair toward the scalp. If the hair is shorter, only a couple of rolls may be needed. A small amount of back-combing will control layers or flyaway hair.

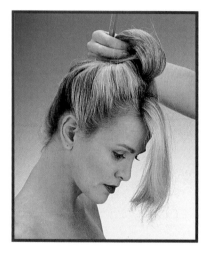

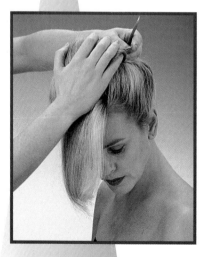

6. With hairpins, secure the rolled hair to the base of the ponytail. (If need be, place an extra hairpin on the other side of the rolled hair.)

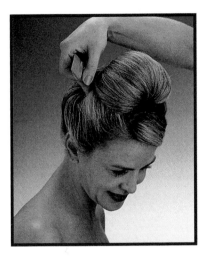

7. Fan the edges of the rolled hair and secure with hairpins inserted so that they catch the scalp hair. Mist lightly with hair spray if extra hold is desired.

8. Bangs or fringe hair may be curled or arranged directionally. Add hair ornaments as desired.

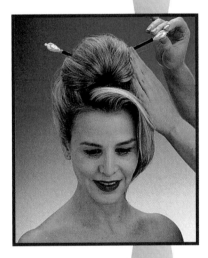

SHIMMERING CASCADES
Double ponytail inversion

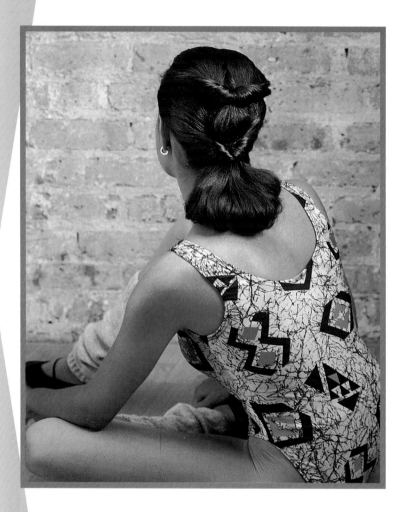

In this design, two ponytails are inverted, one above the other.
The top ponytail flows into the bottom one like a cascading
waterfall. The effect is uniquely attractive and oh, so easy to
achieve!

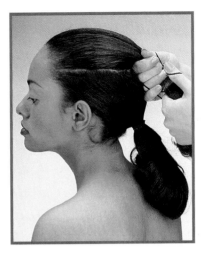

1. Begin by gathering the hair into two equal ponytails, aligned vertically at the back of the head. Fasten each ponytail with a **coated** elastic band.

2. Put the inversion tool through the back of the top ponytail, making sure that the tool passes through the back of the lower ponytail as well.

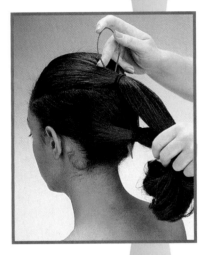

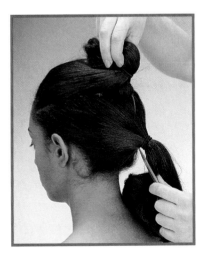

3. Put the top ponytail through the loop of the tool and begin to pull downward.

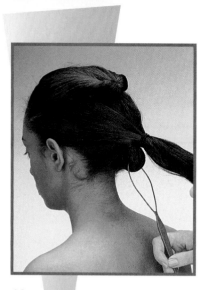

4. Pull the tool all the way through the back of the lower ponytail as well. This enables you to combine the ends of the top ponytail with the ends of the lower ponytail.

5. Repeat the basic inversion technique on the bottom ponytail: Insert the inversion tool behind the elastic band. Pull the ends of the ponytail through the loop, then pull the tool downward through the back of the ponytail.

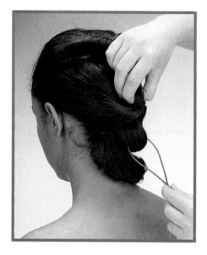

SCULPTURED SOFTNESS
Two-ponytail chignon

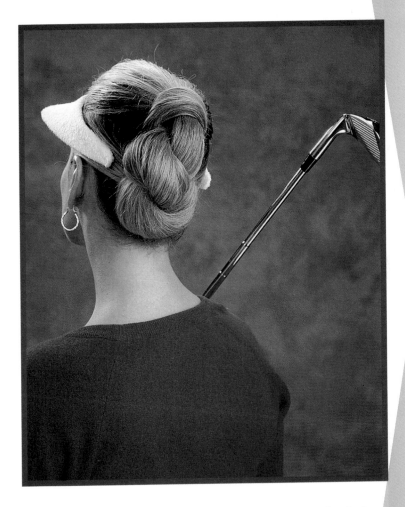

Stunningly beautiful yet simple to create, this smooth, sleek design exemplifies classical elegance. Hair should be at least shoulder length; layered hair can be smoothed back or left to drape softly around the hairline.

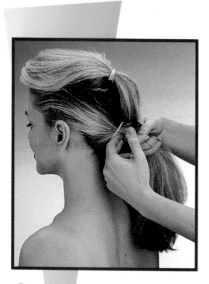

1. Gather hair into two equal ponytails, aligned vertically at the back of the head. Fasten each ponytail with a **coated** elastic band.

2. Holding the top ponytail downward and slightly away from the head, bring the bottom ponytail up along the right side of the top ponytail.

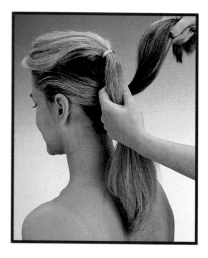

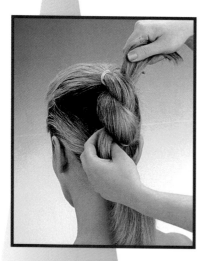

3. Wrap the bottom ponytail over then under the top ponytail. Pull the ends of the bottom ponytail upward so they sit behind the elastic band of the top ponytail.

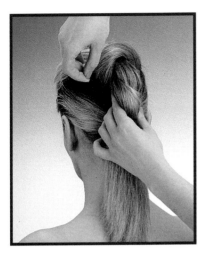

4. Twist the ends of the bottom ponytail around the upper base of the top ponytail, covering the elastic band. Tuck the ends under the crossover area of the two ponytails. Pin in place.

5. Direct the ends from the top ponytail around the base of the lower ponytail, bringing them up toward the right.

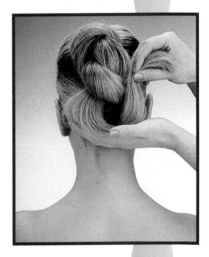

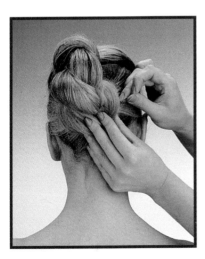

6. Secure the ends with hairpins and mist with hair spray as needed.

SYMMETRICAL PROFUSION
Partial three-strand overbraids

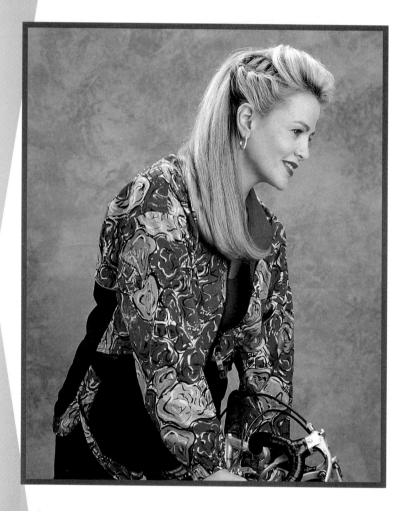

The three-strand overbraid is used to create symmetry in this design. The close contours of the braid on either side contrast with the loose, flowing waves of the rest of the hair.

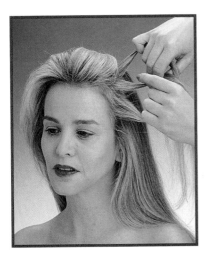

1. Begin on the left side and part the area to be braided. The braid will extend just behind the ear. Section a triangle of hair just off the part and front hairline area. Divide the triangular section into three equal strands.

2. With the left thumb and index finger, grasp the right strand. Cross it over the center strand.

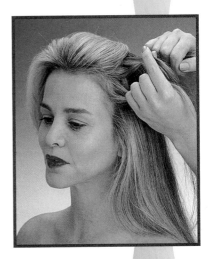

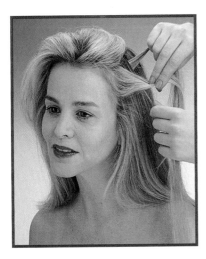

3. Now, with the right thumb and index finger, grasp the left strand and cross it over the center strand.

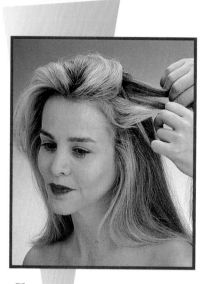

4. Pick up a new section of hair toward the right and join it with the right strand. Cross these combined strands over the center strand.

5. Repeat this procedure along the left side: Pick up a section of hair from the hairline area. Join this with the left strand. Cross these combined strands over the center strand.

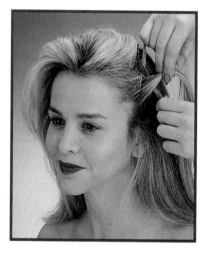

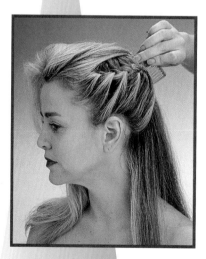

6. Continue the procedure until you reach the area behind the ear. Secure with a decorative comb. Now, perform this three-strand overbraiding technique on the other side of the head and secure with a comb.

CHARMING CONTOURS
Asymmetrical three-strand braid

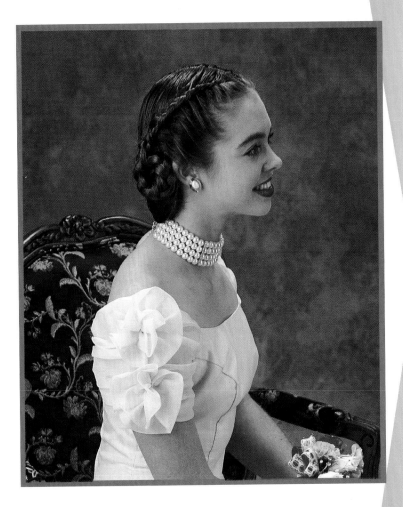

This design is one of the most versatile you'll ever create, as well

as one of the most charming. Asymmetrical three-strand

braiding makes intricate patterns and contours framing the face.

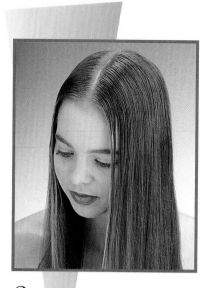

1. Part the hair either down the center or down the side from the front hairline to the nape. Distribute the hair evenly around the head.

2. Part a triangular section at the right front hairline. Direct this section up and back.

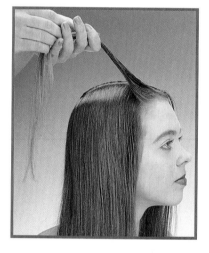

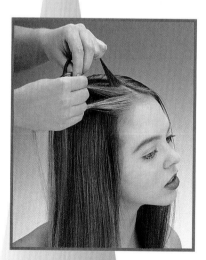

3. Divide the section into three equally sized strands. You're now ready to begin the basic three-strand overbraid.

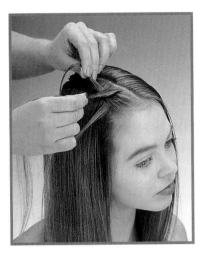

4. With the left thumb and index finger, grasp the right strand and cross it over the center strand. Next, with your right thumb and index finger, grasp the left strand and cross it over the center strand.

5. Before continuing, pick up and add a thin section of hair from the hairline area to the right strand.

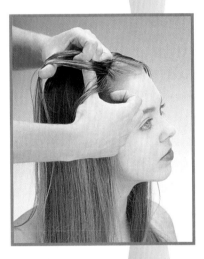

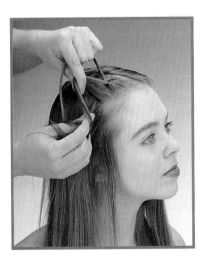

6. With your left thumb and index finger, grasp these joined strands and cross them over the center strand. Continue braiding by crossing the left strand over the center strand.

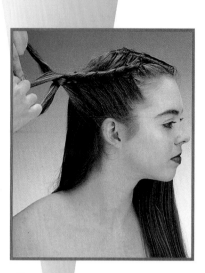

7. Continue braiding back along a diagonal line. (No hair is added to the left strand before crossing it over the center strand—it is only added each time to the right strand before crossing it over the center.)

8. Continue picking up strands from the hairline area along clean, diagonal partings. Add these strands to the right strand until all the hair has been picked up.

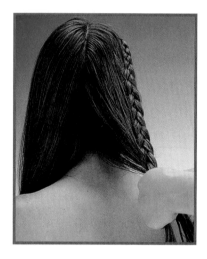

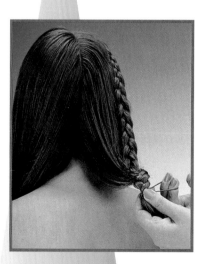

9. Finish the ends in a basic three-strand braid and fasten them with a **coated** elastic band.

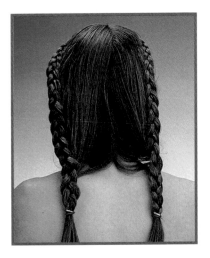

10. Repeat steps 3 through 9 on the left side of the head. Pick up and add the small strands of hair to the left strand as you braid downward.

11. Directing the two braids toward the back of the head, roll the ends of each into a bun just behind the ear.

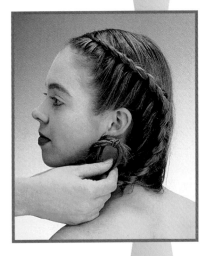

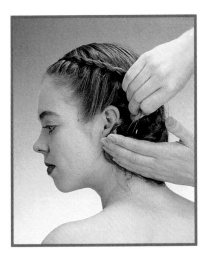

12. Pin in place to secure, and add ornamentation as desired.

CHARMING CONTOURS
First Variation

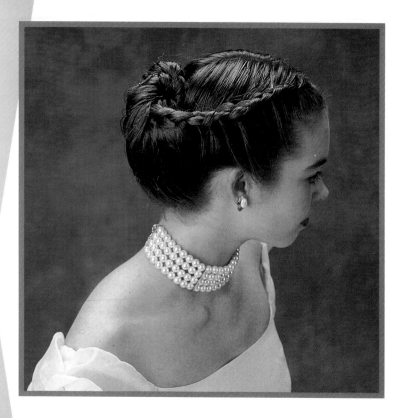

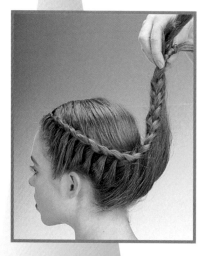

1. Gather the ends of both braids from step 10 of the first design. Lift them up toward the crown. Secure the ends together with a **coated** elastic band.

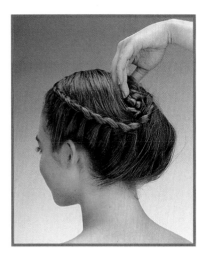

2. Roll the joined ends under at the crown and pin in place. With hairpins, secure both braids to scalp hair. This method of pinning relieves tension on the crown.

Remember...

You can pin or weave decorative ornaments into the braids to design an original look. Be creative!

CHARMING CONTOURS
Second Variation

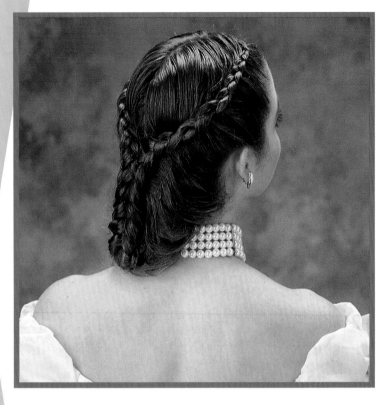

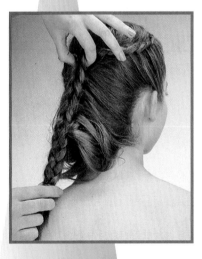

1. Position the two braided sections from step 10 of the first design at the center back of the head. Secure them with bobby pins, edge to edge, to the scalp.

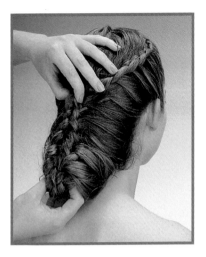

2. Join the ends of the two braids with a **coated** elastic band, then turn the ends under and secure with hairpins.

Remember...

Working with damp hair will give you more control while braiding, but working with dry hair gives a softer effect and greater volume.

ARTFUL WEAVE
Four-strand chain braid

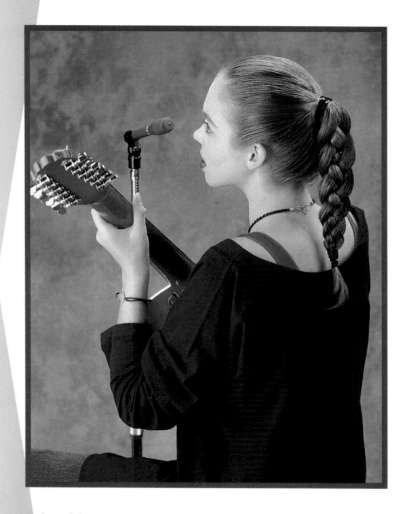

This decorative braid features a woven texture that resembles the jewelry work of a precious-metal chain. The ornate style is created by interlacing four strands and is perfect for longer hair.

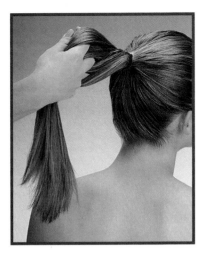

1. Gather the hair smoothly at the crown. Fasten the ponytail with a **coated** elastic band and divide it into four equal strands.

2. To begin the four-strand chain braid technique cross the inside left strand over the inside right strand.

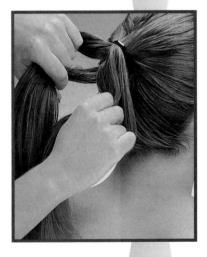

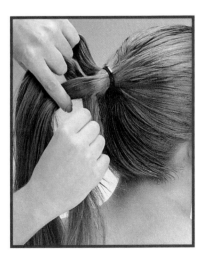

3. Then cross the outside right strand over the inside right strand. (The outside right strand always goes **over** the strand next to it.)

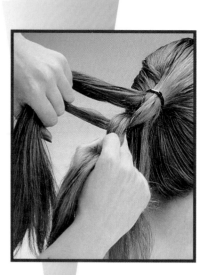

4. Bring this same strand under the next (inside left) strand.

5. Direct the outside left strand under the strand that has just been woven across from the right side. (The left strand always goes **under** the strand next to it.)

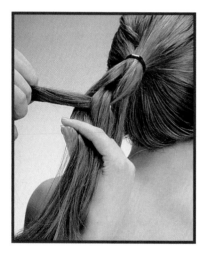

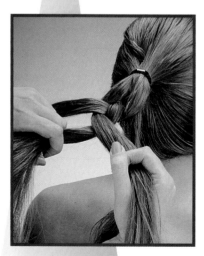

6. Then weave the same strand over the inside right strand.

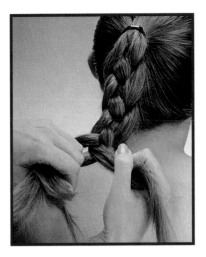

7. Continue weaving the outside strand over and under from one side to the other.

8. Continue weaving to the ends of the hair and fasten them with a **coated** elastic band. Add decorative ornaments.

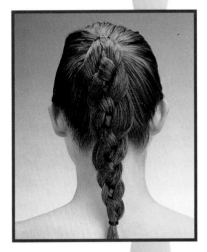

ARTFUL WEAVE
First Variation (with ribbon accent)

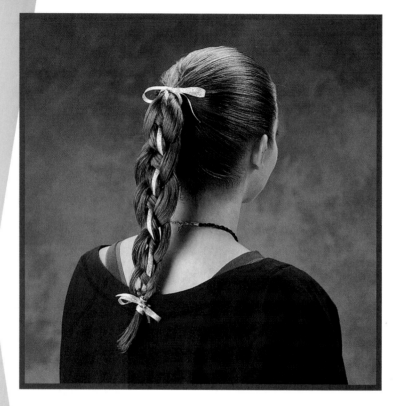

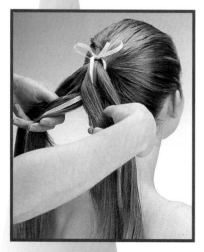

1. Tie a ribbon bow at the base of a ponytail, leaving one long end. Divide the ponytail into four equal strands and let the ribbon trail along the inside right strand. Cross the inside left strand over the inside right strand.

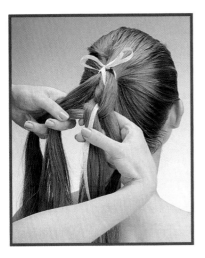

2. Repeat the alternating weave pattern from the first design: Direct the outside right strand over the strand directly next to it and then under the next strand (the one with the ribbon attached).

3. Cross the outside left strand under and then over the inside strands. Do not let the ribbon turn or twist— keep it smooth. Continue chain-braiding to the end of the strands and fasten with a **coated** elastic band.

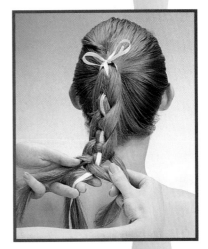

ARTFUL WEAVE
Second Variation (on-the-scalp braid)

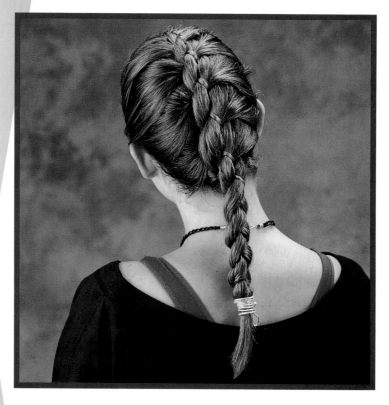

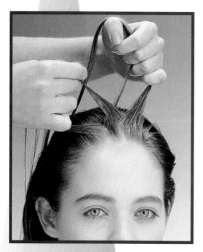

1. Section a triangle of hair from the center front hairline and divide it into four equal strands. Perform the initial four-strand crossovers from the first design: The inside left strand is brought over the inside right strand.

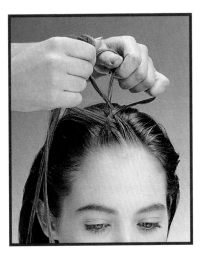

2. The outside right strand is brought over, then under, the inside strands; the outside left strand is brought under, then over, the inside strands.

3. Pick up an elongated section from the hairline to the center of the braiding area and join it to the outside right strand.

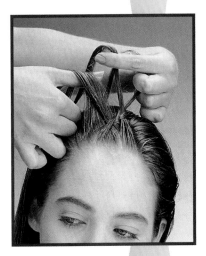

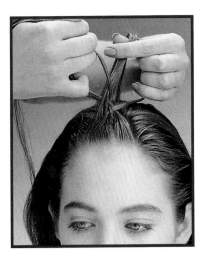

4. Bring these two joined strands together as one and direct them over, then under, the inside strands. Repeat this procedure on the outside left strand.

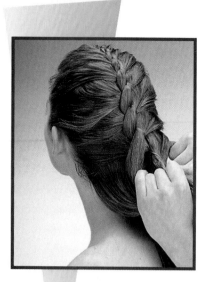

5. Continue until there is no more hair to pick up from the scalp area. When you reach the ends of the hair, fasten with a **coated** elastic band and add ornamentation as desired.

Remember...
Hair spray not only holds the finished design in place, but it also works well in spot areas as you braid.

INTRICATE DELIGHT
Four-strand round braid

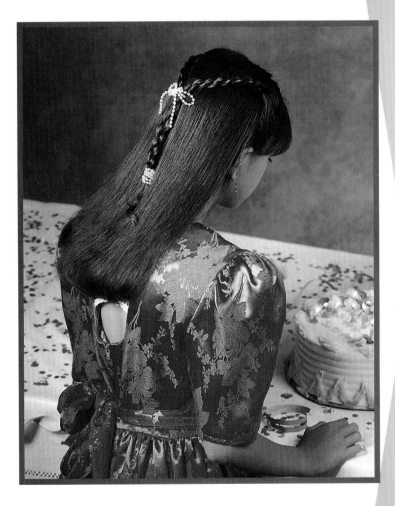

As intricate as this round braid appears, the technique is surprisingly easy. Getting the hang of it is just a matter of synchronizing your hands. You'll soon be on your way to creating many unusual and beautiful designs!

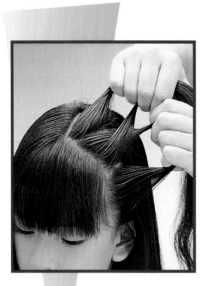

1. Part the hair from the front hairline to the nape. Section a triangle of hair on one side of the part. Divide this section into four equal strands. Cross the inside left strand over the inside right strand.

2. With the right thumb and index finger, grasp and pull the outside left strand under the two inside strands.

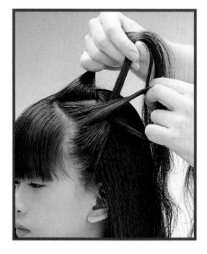

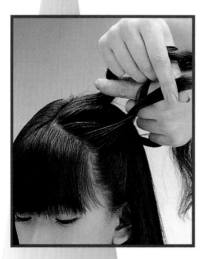

3. Bring that same strand back over the inside right strand. Now, with thumb and index finger of the left hand, grasp the outside right strand from behind the two inside strands.

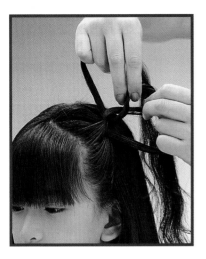

4. Bring the outside right strand under the two inside ones and back over the inside left strand. Continue this until the braid is long enough to reach the center crown area. Clip the braid temporarily.

5. Repeat the four-strand braiding technique on the other side of the head. When you reach the center back, unclip the other four-strand braid and fasten the two together with a **coated** elastic band.

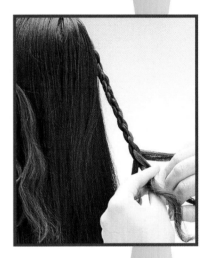

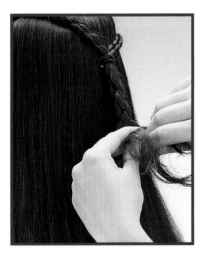

6. Divide the hair that's left over into four equal strands. Repeat the four-strand technique described above and fasten the end with a **coated** elastic band. Add ornamentation as desired.

INTRICATE DELIGHT
Variation

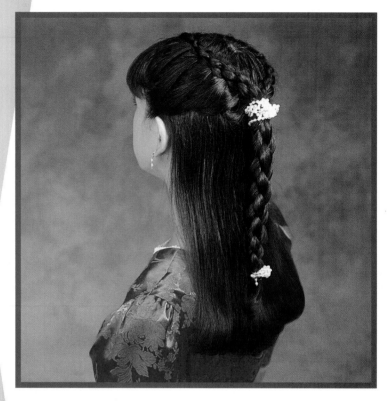

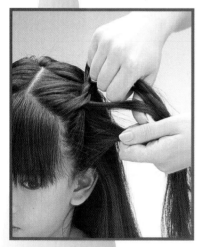

1. Perform the initial crossovers starting on the left side of the head. (Refer to steps 1 through 4 from the first design.) Then pick up hair from along the hairline and add it to the outside left strand.

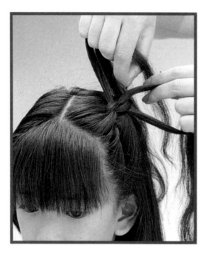

2. With the right hand, reach under the two center strands and grasp the joined outside left strands. Direct these joined strands under the two inside strands and back over the right inside strand.

3. Now, pick up hair from the right side area. Join it to the right strand and repeat the four-strand braiding technique: Cross the pickup strands under the inside strands and back over the left inside strand.

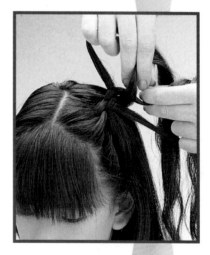

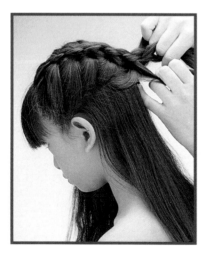

4. Continue braiding, picking up hair through the center back area. At the crown, clip the braid to scalp hair temporarily, then repeat the process on the right side of the head.

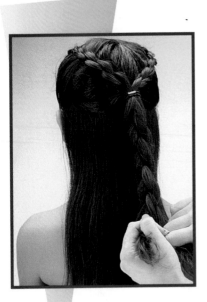

5. Secure the two braids together with a **coated** elastic band. Braid the ponytail ends using the three-strand overbraid technique. Secure the ends with a **coated** elastic band, and add ornaments as desired.

Remember...

You can create an even more intricate style by using the four-strand braiding technique on the joined ponytail ends from step 5.